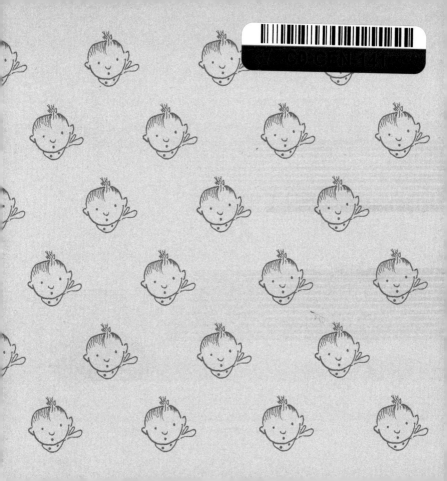

for . . . .

· baby ·

by

Lauren White

Sourcebooks, Inc.
Naperville, IL

BABIES CREATE...

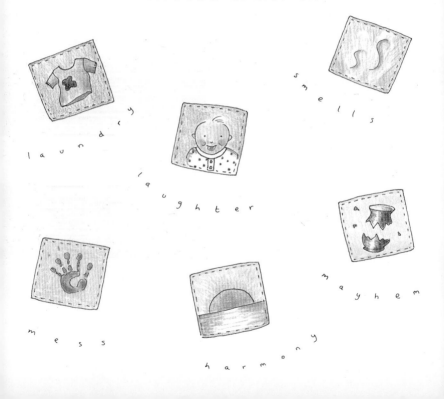

laundry

smells

laughter

mess

harmony

mayhem

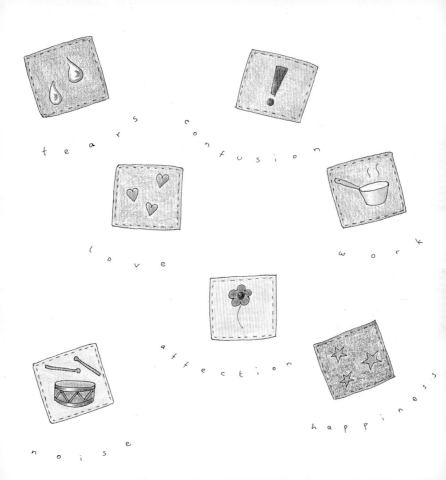

tears confusion

love work

affection

noise happiness

when I grow up I want to be an

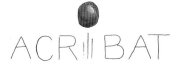

ACR BAT

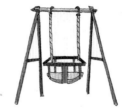

baby's first lesson

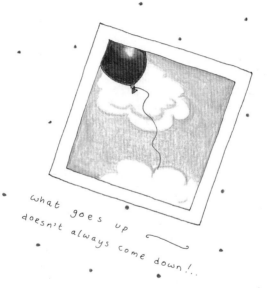

what goes up
doesn't always come down!...

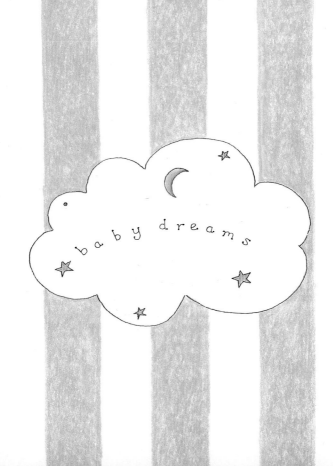

baby dreams

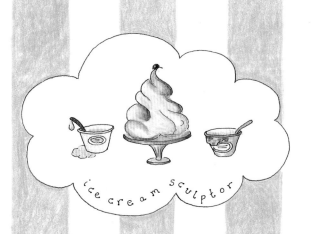

ice cream sculptor

a day in the life....

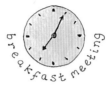

breakfast meeting

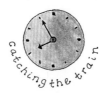

catching the train

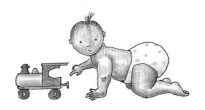

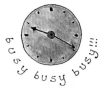

busy busy busy!!!

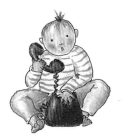

working lunch

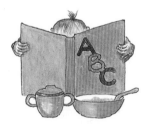

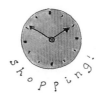

shopping!

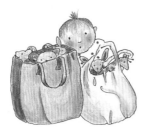

siesta

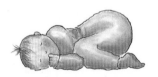

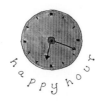

happy hour

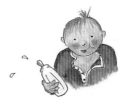

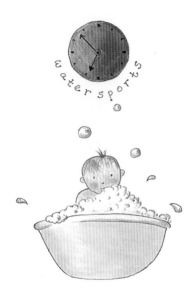

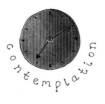

contemplation

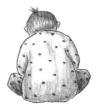

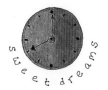

sweet dreams

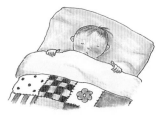

when I grow up I want to be a

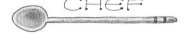

CHEF

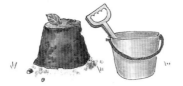

baby's first smile

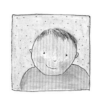

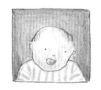

♡ b a b y t a l e n t s № 1 ♡

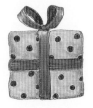

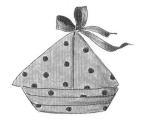

to love the wrapping!

baby's first lesson

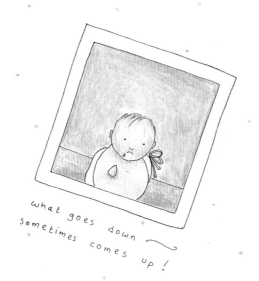

what goes down
sometimes comes up!

when I grow up I want to be a

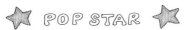 POP STAR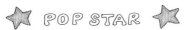

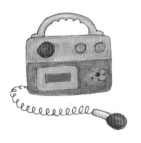

skin as soft as a . . . .

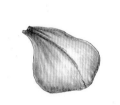

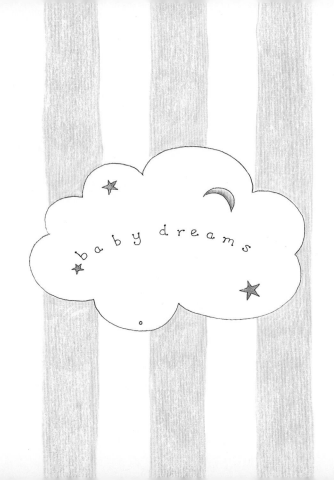

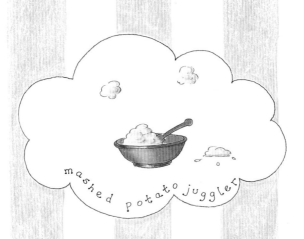

mashed potato juggler

baby's first lesson

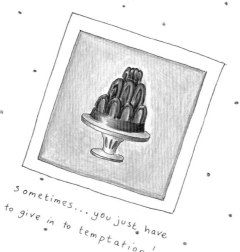

Sometimes... you just have to give in to temptation!

when I grow up I want to be a

SOCIALITE

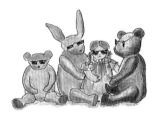

♡ b a b y   t a l e n t s   №2 ♡

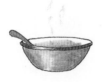

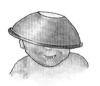

to thoroughly enjoy dinner!

baby's first lesson

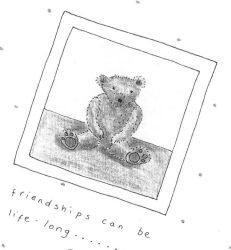

friendships can be

life-long . . . .

NAMING BABY

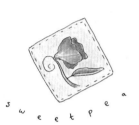

sweet pea

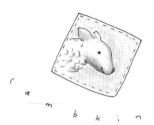

lambkin

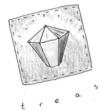

treasure

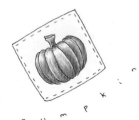

pumpkin

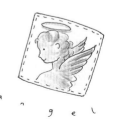

angel

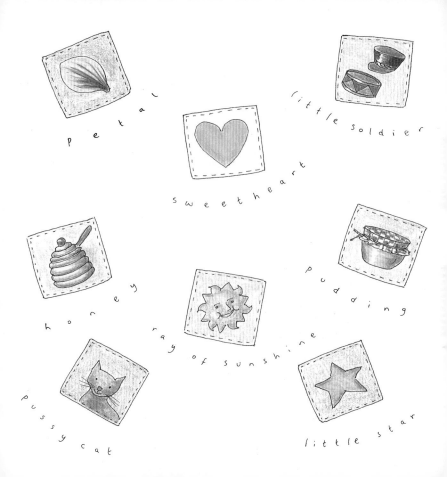

petal

little soldier

sweetheart

honey

ray of sunshine

pudding

pussy cat

little star

when I grow up I want to be an

INTERIOR DESIGNER

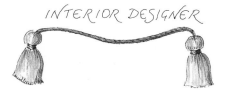

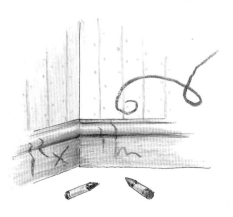

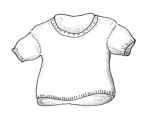

· b e f o r e ·

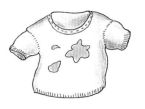

· a f t e r ·

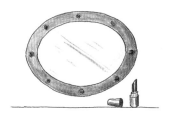

· b e f o r e ·

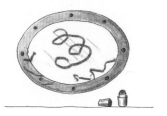

· a f t e r ·

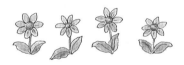

. b e f o r e .

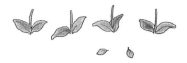

after

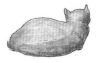

· be o re ·

f

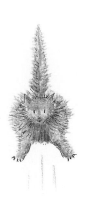

· after ·

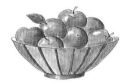

. b e f o r e .

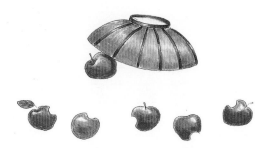

after

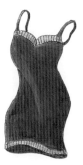

· b e x o r e ·

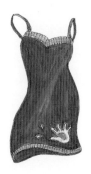

. a s t e r .

Oops!

when I grow up I want to be a

M·A·T·H·E·M·A·T·I·C·I·A·N

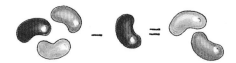

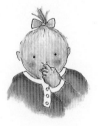

♡ b a b y   t a l e n t s   № 3 ♡

to touch your nose...

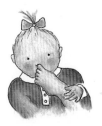

...with your toes!

baby's first friend

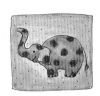

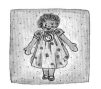

when I grow up I want to be a

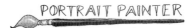 PORTRAIT PAINTER

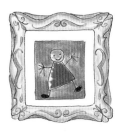

a smile like......

when I grow up I want to be an

EXPLORER

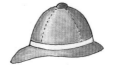

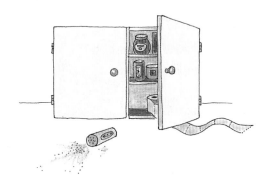

♡ b a b y t a l e n t s Nº4 ♡

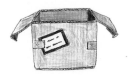

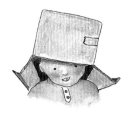

to find a cardboard box interesting...

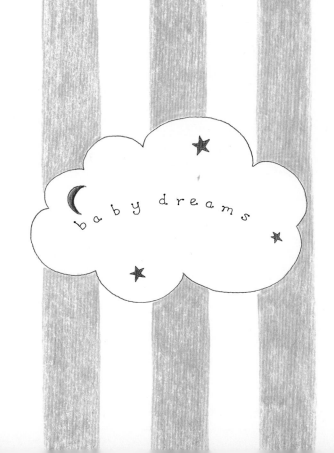

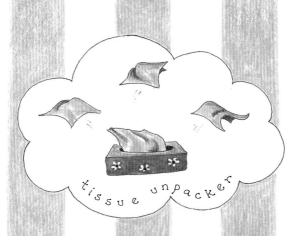

tissue unpacker

baby's first lesson

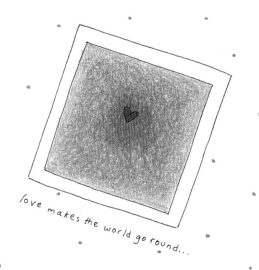

love makes the world go round...

when I grow up I want to be a

DOCTOR

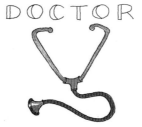

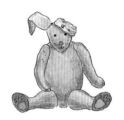

♡ b a b y t a l e n t s №5 ♡

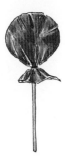

not to hide emotions!

eyes like bright little....

when I grow up I want to be an

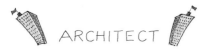

ARCHITECT

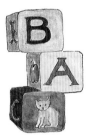

♡ b a b y t a l e n t s №6 ♡

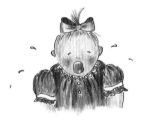

perfect timing!

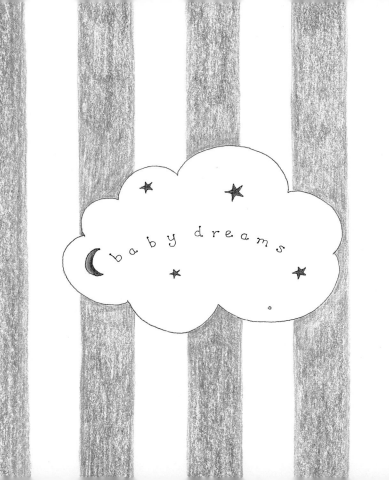

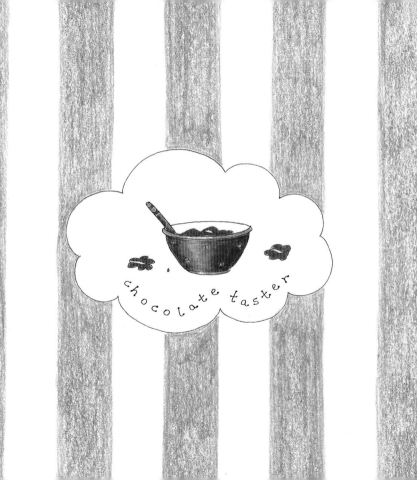

chocolate taster

baby's first tooth

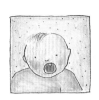
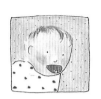

when I grow up I want to be a

 ZOO KEEPER

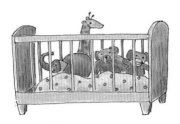

♡ b a b y t a l e n t s №7 ♡

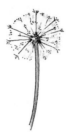

the ability to be fascinated
by a little bit of fluff...

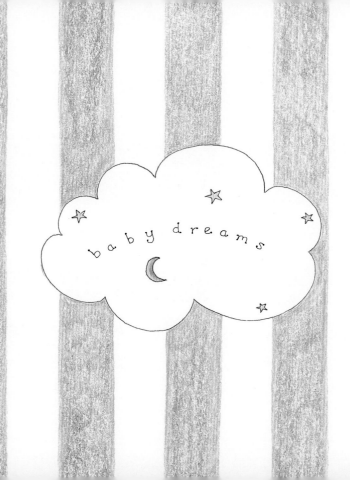

baby dreams

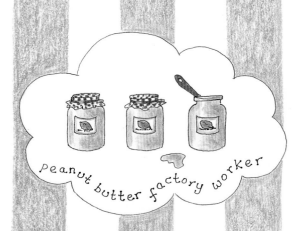

peanut butter factory worker

laughter that tinkles like little.....

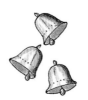

when I grow up I want to be a

SECRET AGENT

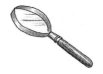

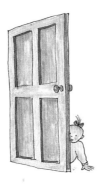

♡ b a b y   t a l e n t s   №8 ♡

to inspire more love than anything on earth

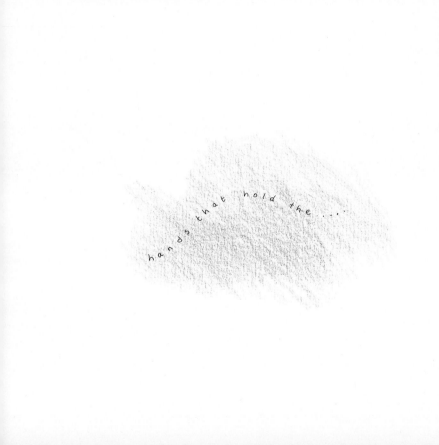

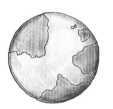

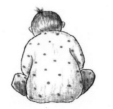

"Adding a sprinkling of magic to the everyday"... is how Lauren White describes her original style of drawing. Born and brought up in the Bedfordshire village of Cranfield, she studied fine art in Hull and London before returning to Bedfordshire to work as resident illustrator for a local wildlife trust. She loves playing the piano, walking her dog, Jack and carries a sketchbook everywhere she goes. She lives with her partner, Michael, and describes herself as having an astonishing collection of marbles and a wicked sense of humour. Lauren's designs for Hotchpotch greetings cards are sold around the world and in this book she continues to refine her distinctive style which "celebrates the simple things in life."

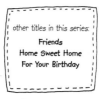

other titles in this series:

Friends
Home Sweet Home
For Your Birthday

Published in 2000 by
Sourcebooks, Inc
1935 Brookdale Road, Suite 139
Naperville IL 60563

Text & Illustrations © Lauren White 2000
Printed and bound in China

MQ 10 9 8 7 6 5 4 3 2 1

ISBN: 1-57071-520-3

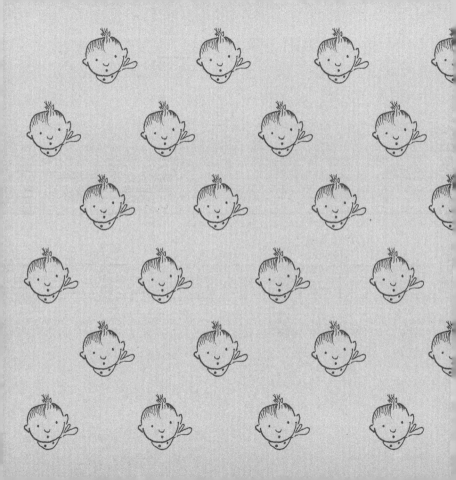